Coconut Oil: A Step-By-Step

Guide for Beginners Including Easy Recipes

Disclaimer

The author has tried to be an authentic source of the information provided in this report. However, the author does not oppose the additional information available over the internet. The objective of providing different benefits, step-by-step guidelines of coconut oil, and its recipes is to enable readers to get an idea of the usefulness of coconut oil for culinary purposes and various other uses. The information included in this book cannot be compared with the coconut oil recipes provided in other books. All readers can seek further help through additional sources of information.

Ignoring any of the guidelines or not following the essential information available in this book may not give you the exact result. Therefore, the author is not responsible for such negligence.

Table of Contents

Why Should You Read This Book?

Almond oil, olive oil, jojoba oil, coconut oil, and mustard oil are some of the most common choices to pick the oil you like the most. But why choose coconut oil? What is so good about it that other kinds of oil do not have? Tropics call it the magical oil because of its unique properties in terms of providing skin and health benefits, and culinary variations.

By reading this book, you will learn the truth behind the high demand of coconut oil. Backed by millions of benefits, this book will guide you how to incorporate the use of coconut oil in your daily use, as well as in your diet. Additionally, it is considered a special ingredient in different recipes. Read on the recipes provided in this book, and you will learn how to incorporate the same to your diet.

To specify it even further, this book comprises of the following valuable information:

a. Information about coconut oil
b. Various benefits of coconut oil
c. How to use coconut oil according to different situations
d. Breakfast, lunch, dinner, and appetizer recipes in which coconut oil is the main ingredient

CHAPTER 1

Coconut Oil – The Miracle Oil

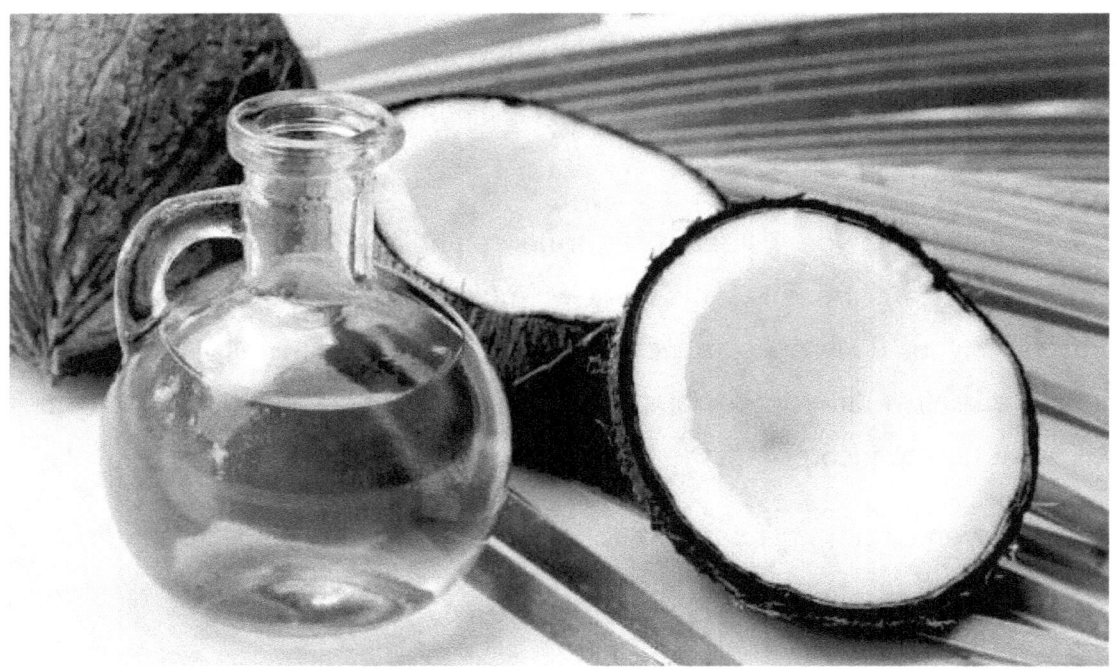

Are you anxious to explore why people from tropical regions cannot imagine living without coconuts? Since coconuts have been considered daily yet, special food for them, they use it for a large number of reasons. So, what is the miracle in coconut oil? Simply put, this oil is unique among all other oils. This is one of the reasons why it has become so popular all around the world.

What makes coconut oil stand out from other oils is the unique level of fat molecules present in it. Sounds too technical? Let's look at it in detail.

All oils and fats contain fat molecules, which are actually called fatty acids or triglycerides. These fatty acids are divided into 3 categories, i.e. Long-Chain Triglycerides (LCT), Medium-Chain Triglycerides (MCT), and Short-Chain Triglycerides (SCT).

The secret behind high demand of coconut oil reveals here: The size of the triglycerides in oil is what matters the most in terms of nutrition and healing powers. Considering this, the majority of oils consist of LCT. However, coconut oil is composed of MCT, which can be absorbed and digested in the body easily as compared to LCT and SCT. However, all this does not end here. This unique form of fatty acids present in coconut oil provides instant energy to the body, and fasters the healing process.

CHAPTER 2: Coconut Oil for Hair Care

As you search for numerous hair treatment products in the market, you will notice that there are many, but there are only a few which are really worth buying. Coconut oil is one of them. Known as the natural source of vitamins for your hair, you can avail the maximum hair care benefits from coconut oil.

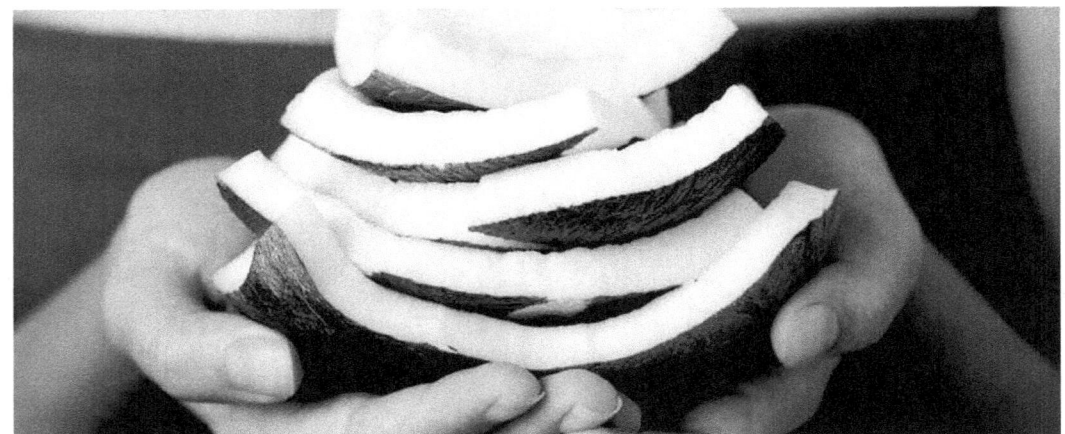

Coconut Oil for Hair Growth

Filled with moisturizing properties, coconut oil moisturizes the scalp too. It moisturizes it, and aids in hair growth. Since dead and dry skin cells can clog the hair follicles, and stop hair growth, applying coconut oil to your scalp can help you get healthy hair follicles. As a result, it boosts the hair growth process.

Coconut Oil for Dandruff Treatment

Tired of fighting with dandruff? Learn what coconut oil can do to your hair, and you will never stop using it! This is especially true if you want to get rid of hair dandruff.

Basically, dandruff can also be said as fungal infection of hair. The use of coconut oil is ideal here because it is anti-fungal oil, which is considered ideal for hair dandruff treatment.

Coconut Oil for Hair Damage

Your hair may have damaged even before you notice them. This is mainly because of various factors, for instance, pollution, overuse of heated tools, perms, bleaching, or dyeing. Overtime, your hair can have split ends, leading to breakage. Rather than using expensive products full of chemicals, you can use coconut oil to moisturize the damaged surface of your hair. If done regularly, your hair can recover from this damage quickly.

How to Use Coconut Oil for Hair Care

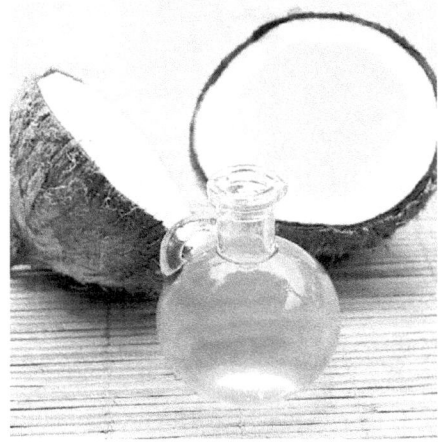

Whether you are looking for the right solution to repair the hair damage, or you want to get rid of hair dandruff, following the below-mentioned steps will help you use coconut oil in the most beneficial way:

1. Place a tablespoon of coconut oil into your hand. Rub both the hands together, so that the coconut oil can be warmed.
2. Now, start applying from your scalp to the hair tips. Make sure you cover all the scalp as well as hair strands with the oil. Once this is done, massage for 15 minutes.
3. Wait for at least an hour so that coconut oil can be absorbed well.
4. Now, wash your hair the way you do till you feel that the oil is completely removed from your hair.

For best results, repeat this hair oil treatment once or twice a week.

CHAPTER 3: Coconut Oil for Skin Care

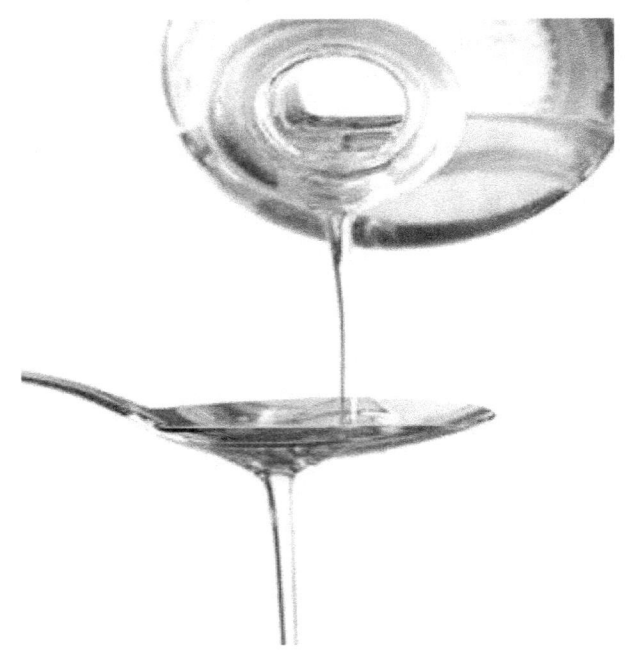

Coconut Oil as Skin Moisturizer

Coconut oil is considered an extremely effective treatment for dry skin. This natural oil is rich in Vitamin E, and therefore, it reduces skin flaking, and clears any skin blockages.

Since applying the right moisturizer to your skin is the primary thing required to avoid getting wrinkles before you start aging, coconut oil has that magic that can help you with this. By inhibiting face wrinkling, the moisturizer within coconut oil aids in enhancing skin youth.

How to Use Coconut Oil to Moisturize Your Skin

1. Before applying coconut oil on your skin, perform a small skin test to know if your skin is not allergic to coconut oil.
2. After that, wash your face with a mild cleanser, and dry it with a clean cloth.
3. Apply a bit of coconut oil on your face and neck, and spread it evenly, in circular motions. Leave it overnight so that it is absorbed well into your skin

Coconut Oil to Fight Skin Infection

The level of Vitamin E present in coconut oil fights skin infections. Some of these include acne, eczema, dermatitis, and psoriasis.

How to Use Coconut Oil to Fight Infection

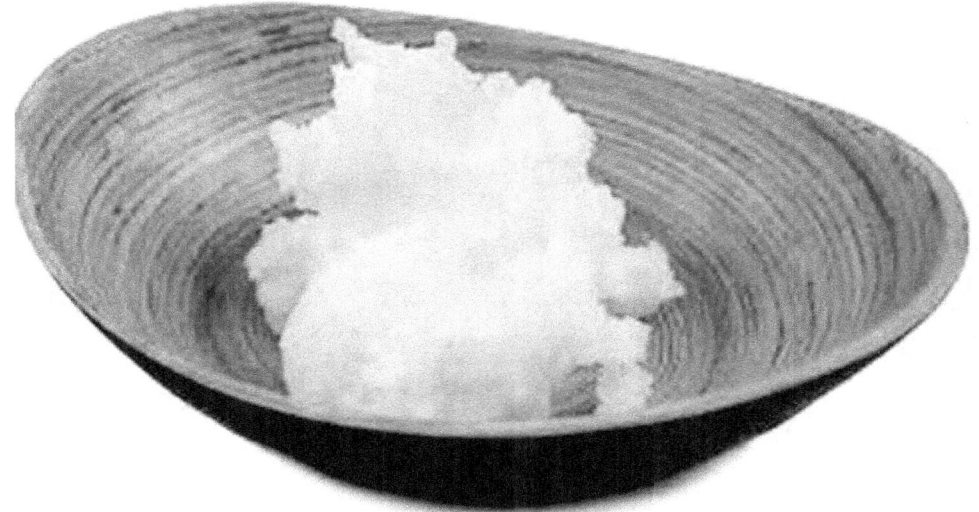

Melt the coconut oil till it gets naturally warm. Take a drop of it and apply gently on the affected area of your skin. Make sure that the oil is well-absorbed.

Coconut Oil for Eye Area

Only a few drops of coconut oil can do wonders to your eye area. If you have wrinkles under your eyes, or you simply do not want to have them at all, applying coconut oil on the same area of skin, and leaving it overnight can give you ever-young eyes.

How to Use Coconut Oil to Avoid Wrinkles

Wash your face with a mild soap or face wash. Apply a bit of coconut oil on the eye area. Massage gently. Leave it there overnight.

CHAPTER 4: Coconut Oil as Medicine

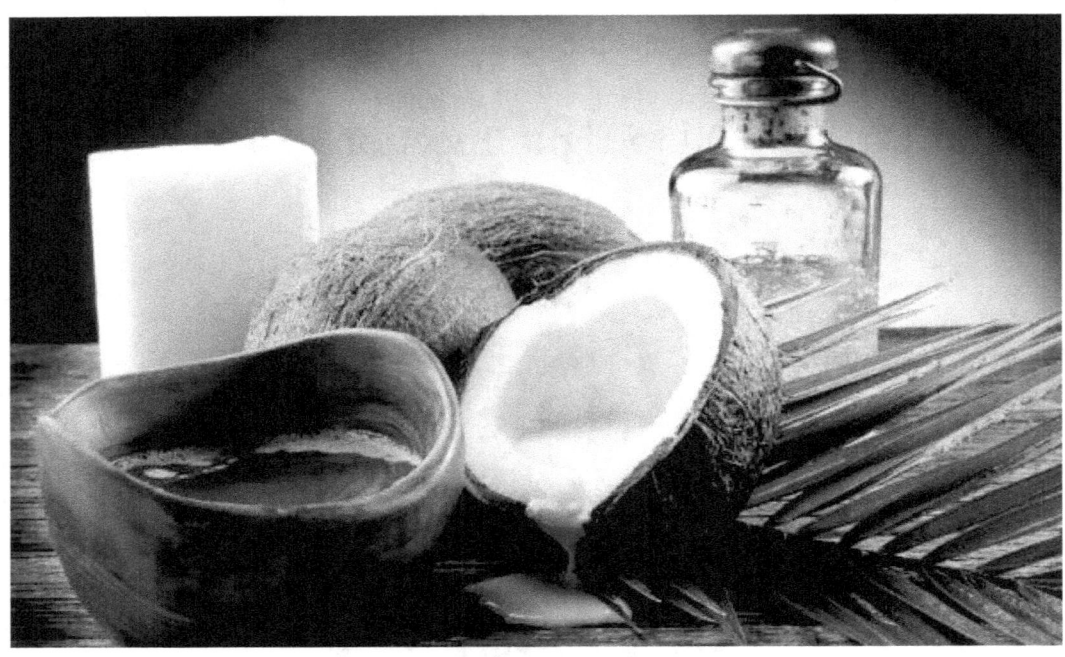

Coconut Oil as Antibiotic

According to health professionals, coconut oil contains numerous antibacterial components that other kinds of oils do not. For example, coconut oil contains lauric acid, the acid that is considered one of the most powerful negative bacteria and virus destroyer. This makes coconut oil worth using, as it also destroys various other viruses, such as, HIV, herpes, influenza virus, measles, giardia lamblia, and some pathogenic bacteria.

Coconut Oil for Immune System

As discussed above, the secret ingredient of coconut oil, i.e. lauric acid is all that provides you exceptional health benefits of using coconut oil. This applies well for your immune system too. Along with promoting heart health, coconut oil helps you lower cholesterol, and speed up your metabolism, leading to an overall boost in your immune system.

Coconut Oil for Healing and Repairing Tissues

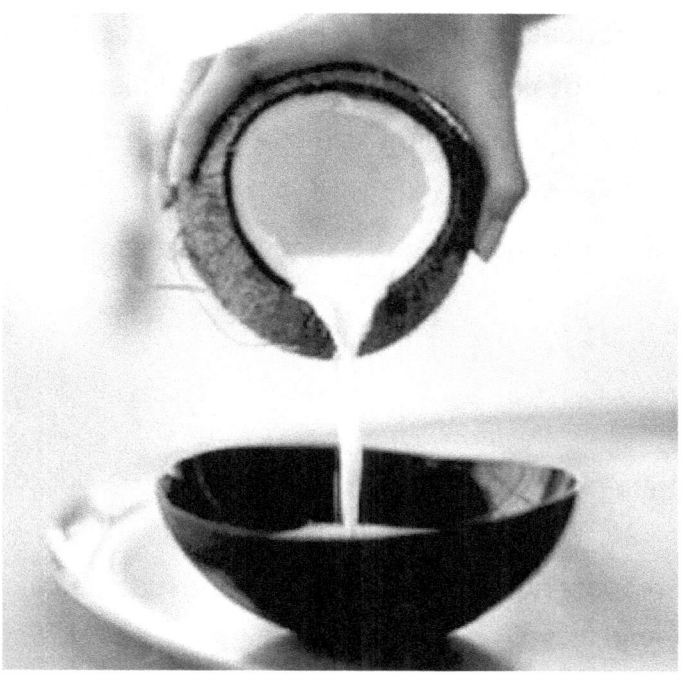

There are various skin conditions that result in dryness, harshness, and rashes in the skin. This is when the skin tissues need the most of healing and repairing. Applying coconut oil to the affected areas of skin helps in healing rashes, dryness, and itching. As a result, it smoothes skin and aids in repairing of skin tissues.

Coconut Oil for Hypertension

Hypertension (high blood pressure) is a medical condition that has affected millions of people. Though taking medicines prescribed by your doctor should be considered the primary way to deal with it, it is equally important to add natural and essential oils to your diet that aid in lowering the level of blood pressure.

Coconut oil is one of those essential oils that will help you control your blood pressure as it contains omega-3 fatty acids that are considered better to lower blood pressure as compared to vegetable oils.

Coconut Oil for Diabetes

Though not a lot of information is known in terms of coconut oil usage for Type 1 diabetes patients, one thing is confirmed. Having a good diet that consists of coconut oil rather than other fats plays a significant role in protecting the body against the insulin resistance. Along with this, coconut oil provides many other benefits to improve health. However, the amount of coconut oil to be incorporated in diet depends on what your doctor recommends.

Coconut Oil for Eczema

Due to its antibacterial properties, coconut oil is considered one of the effective oils for the treatment of eczema. When the skin becomes itchy, and dry with visible scars and rashes, applying pure coconut oil on these eczema patches soothes the skin, and removes the dryness with the help of its natural moisture.

How to Use Coconut Oil as Medicine

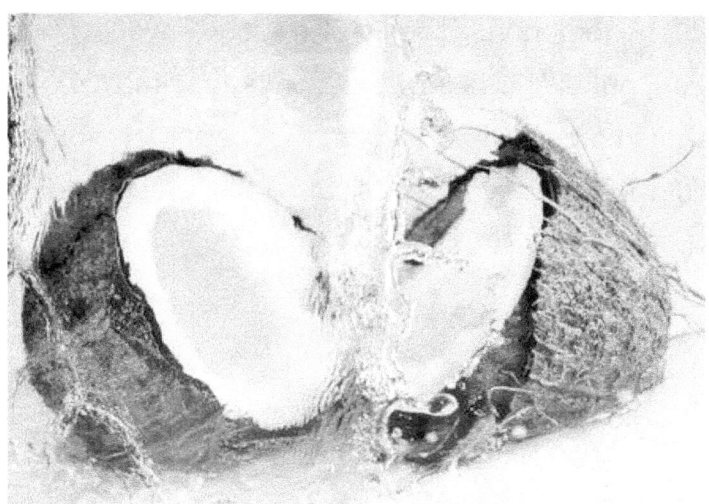

By now, you must have got a clear idea of the different medicinal uses of coconut oil. Since each medical condition requires a different usage of coconut oil, there are different methods to treat each medical condition.

To use coconut oil externally, you can apply a few drops of coconut oil on the affected skin, and massage it gently. Do not rinse it immediately with water, as this may hinder with its effectiveness. For this reason, it is recommended that you should apply coconut oil to your skin before going to bed. Since the oil stays there on the skin, and is absorbed overnight, it may provide you better results.

CHAPTER 5: Coconut Oil for Stress Relief

Stress is a common phenomenon, especially in today's world where everyone is faced with tough competition, but did you know that your stress may lead you to various health conditions which should actually be avoided? Caring for your mental health is as important as doing the same for your physical health. Here, adding coconut oil to your daily routine can help you relieve stress.

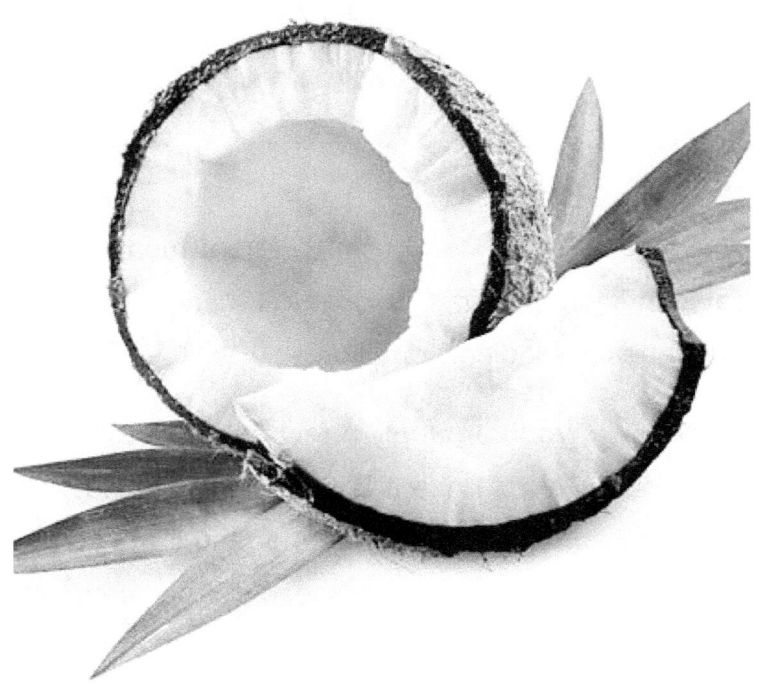

Coconut Oil for Mental Fatigue and Migraine

Migraine can be one of the causes of mental fatigue due to lack of sleep. Though many people consume aspirin as suggested by their doctor, they can also go for a natural remedy. Coconut oil is one of the natural remedies that not only relieves mental fatigue, its aroma stays for longer which soothes the mind.

Coconut Oil for Anxiety and Depression

Sometimes all your head needs is a bit of coconut oil massage. When applied to your hair and scalp in circular motion, it provides a feeling of relaxation and positivity. As a result, it is considered effective in terms of getting rid of anxiety and depression.

Coconut Oil for Heart Health

Though coconut oil contains saturated fats, it is important to know that if taken a specific proportion of coconut oil as suggested by a health professional, coconut oil can actually be good for your heart.

With healthy fat properties, coconut oil helps you avoid heart attack or stroke. Furthermore, it promotes cardiovascular health, and maintains healthy levels of cholesterol within your body.

How to Use Coconut Oil for Stress Relief

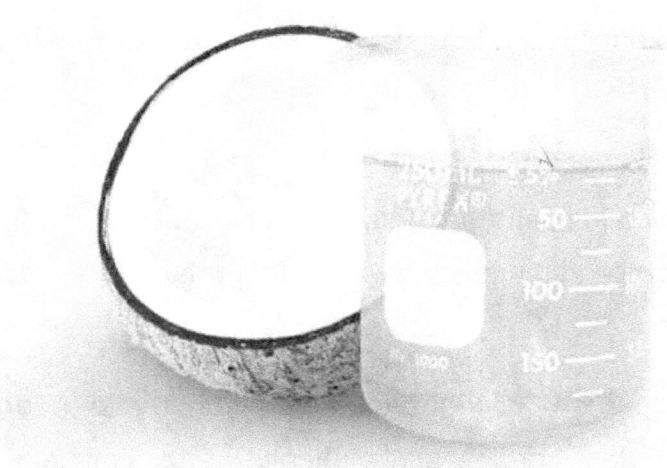

To relieve stress, there are two ways to use coconut oil:

1. Incorporate it into your daily diet. For instance, rather than using any other oil in cooking, make use of coconut oil. Here, you need to add the same quantity of oil as you used to use the other oil in cooking.
2. Use coconut oil as a hair tonic. Pour some of it in your palm, rub both hands to make it warmer, and then apply to your scalp. Massage gently. This way, you will notice that you are no more feeling tired.

CHAPTER 6: Coconut Oil for Anti-Aging

Why should you use expensive anti-wrinkle creams when you have something natural and inexpensive right in your kitchen cabinet? Yes, we are talking about coconut oil. Free from harsh chemicals which are mostly present in anti-aging products, coconut oil can provide your skin with even better results.

Coconut Oil for Wrinkles

Since coconut oil is good for skin, it has the same beneficial properties that help you remove wrinkles from your skin. If applied to face as a natural moisturizer on a daily basis, you can delay the aging process of your skin, turning it into well-nourished and young-looking skin.

Coconut Oil for Dark Spots

If dark spots are not in your genes, then age may be one of the reasons of getting dark spots on your skin. However, it may also be premature aging. Again, coconut oil can be used here as the magic oil to reduce your dark spots. Since it does not contain any chemicals, it can work directly to lighten your dark spots. However, make sure you use it regularly.

How to Use Coconut Oil to Fight Anti-Aging

Since both the wrinkles and dark spots are skin conditions, you can get rid of them by using coconut oil externally. If you want to ensure that your skin remains young, apply a few drops of coconut oil into your face and neck, massage slowly, and sleep well. Repeat this daily, and see the result.

A similar procedure applies to reduce aging spots except one thing, i.e. you need to apply a bit of coconut oil only on the dark spots. Repeat this for several days before going to bed, and notice the change.

CHAPTER 7: Coconut Oil for Weight Loss

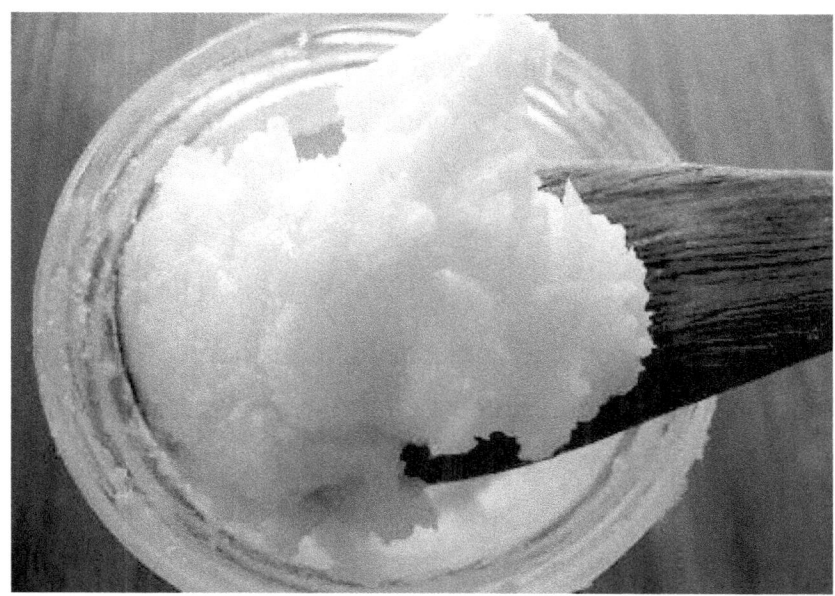

It definitely seems weird to hear about the oil that aids in weight loss instead of weight gain. However, various research studies have proven this fact true! Read on to know how using coconut oil can actually help you lose weight.

The Advantage of Fats Present in Coconut Oil

Coconut oil contains low calories as compared to other oils. Additionally, what differentiates it from other these oils is the that that it does not convert fat to carbohydrates. As it comprises of medium chain fatty acids, the fats absorbed by the body are directly utilized by cells, transforming into energy rather than weight gain.

Burns fat

The medium chain fatty acids promote fat oxidation by burning stored fats of the body. This way, you are able to shed those extra pounds easily.

Increases Metabolism

Weight loss has a lot to do with the thyroid function of your body. Coconut oil aids in improving the same. This leads to the production of a higher level of thyroxin, i.e. your body's accelerator. This way, your body tends to produce more energy, even while you are resting. The result? Your body starts losing weight!

Burns Calories

Your body requires something that consists of thermogenic properties to burn extra calories. Coconut oil has the same property that aids in weight loss. When calories are burnt, your body becomes more active and warm.

Suppresses Appetite

This depends entirely on how you consume coconut oil. If you take it before meals, coconut oil will reduce your appetite as you may feel fuller. As a result, you will eat less. Making it a habit will help you lose weight within a couple of weeks.

How to Use Coconut Oil for Weight Loss

You can use coconut oil while cooking healthy food of your choice. Likewise, you can also top salads with it. However, the quantity of coconut oil should be something you need to consider. This mainly depends on your own body weight. Have a look below to see how much of coconut oil you should be consuming per day:

a. 2 tablespoons if you have over 34 kg weight
b. 2.5 tablespoons if you have over 45 kg weight
c. 3 tablespoons if you have over 57 kg weight

Though this is how it has been calculated according to your weight, you can have the amount of coconut oil depending on what your dietitian has suggested you.

It can easily be digested. So, you can take it 30 minutes before your meal. Also, remember that you need to continue your workout schedule even if you are consuming coconut oil.

CHAPTER 8: Misconceptions Related to the Use of Coconut Oil

When it comes to getting knowledge about various foods, their benefits, and risks, we mostly rely on what others say. However, not all this information absorbed by our minds is authentic. For this reason, one should always go for scientific research, but what about the misconceptions about something you have been hearing for years? Those misconceptions remain myths. However, it is important to identify the true facts.

Likewise, when you hear about the uses of coconut oil, there are high chances that you will come across the following misconceptions about it. However, the truth may completely be opposite.

Misconception No. 1

Coconut oil is composed of saturated fats. These fats raise cholesterol level. Additionally, they increase the risk of having a heart attack.

Fact

Most people are still unaware of the fact that cholesterol is categorized into two different types, i.e. the good one, and the bad one. So, when there is a discussion about the level of saturated fats in coconut oil, this simply means that it is all about High Density Lipoprotiens (HDL) cholesterol.

Coconut oil raises this type of cholesterol, which is actually healthy. Furthermore, HDL cholesterol raises the Low Density Lipoprotiens (LDL) cholesterol (bad cholesterol). This way, it helps clean the blocked arteries, and protects the heart.

Misconception No.2

The level of saturated fats in coconut oil contributes in weight gain, leading to obesity.

Fact

These saturated fats are actually called medium chain fatty acids. These fats increase the metabolism rate of the body. This means that your body tends to consume more energy, leading to burning more fats. Furthermore, taking the prescribed amount of coconut oil will help you lose weight.

Misconception No. 3

Coconut oil irritates the skin

Fact

This is something which is completely opposite for coconut oil. This is because coconut oil actually soothes the skin. This is true even if your skin is severely damaged from sun exposure, or if you have any skin disease. For instance, if you have got an insect sting, allergy, bruises, or a reaction of any drug, coconut oil can be the best natural source to soothe your skin.

Even if you have got wounds, you can get maximum advantage of this by utilizing the anti-microbial properties of this amazing coconut oil.

Misconception No. 4

Coconut oil is sweet, but not healthy for diabetics

Fact

First of all, this oil is not sweet. It simply cannot be because it definitely does not consist of any glucose. How it controls diabetes is a commonly asked question. It promotes insulin secretion from pancreas. This is how coconut oil has the properties to control diabetes. Furthermore, research reveals that using coconut oil on a regular basis may reduce the chance of having diabetes. However, you should consult your doctor before adding it to your daily routine.

Chapter 9: Coconut Oil Recipes

Too boring to add coconut oil in the same dishes again and again? Even if you realize the health benefits of this magic oil, you still need something exciting to start off your day with. The following recipes will help you make the most of coconut oil:

Breakfast Recipes

Coconut Cookies with Almonds and Chocolate Chips

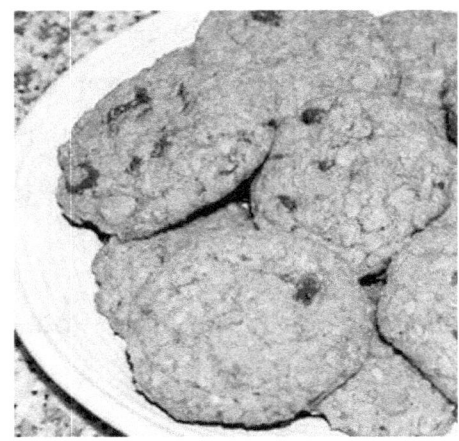

Ingredients

Organic oats (processed): 2 ½ cups

Organic butter (softened): ½ cup

Coconut oil (organic): ½ cup

Brown sugar (organic): 1 cup

Granulated sugar (organic): 1 cup

Eggs: 2

Pure vanilla: 1 teaspoon

Whole wheat flour: 1 cup

Unbleached flour: 1 cup

Baking powder: 1 teaspoon

Shredded (organic) coconut: 1 cup

Almonds (chopped/whole): 1 cup

Chocolate chips: 2 cups

Directions

1. Take a blender or a food processor, and place oats in it. Process them till they have turned into smaller pieces. Make sure not to process them too much and avoid turning them into fine flour.

2. Now, preheat your oven to a temperature of 375 degrees.

3. Take a medium-sized bowl, and pour coconut oil and butter in it. Mix both the ingredients well till they are turned into a smooth cream. Now, add both kinds of sugar, and beat the mixture until fluffy. Beat in vanilla and eggs. When this is done, set this bowl aside.

4. Now that you are left with dry ingredients, mix all of them together. Add this dry mixture to the creamed mixture. Combine this mixture well. After that, add chocolate chips, almonds, and coconut in it, and mix well. The dough for coconut cookies is ready.

5. Roll the dough into small balls, and place them on the cookie sheets. Bake them in the heated oven for about 6 minutes. Flatten them with spatula. Now, bake them for 5 more minutes.

6. When this is done, remove the cookies from the oven, and let them cool on the pan for about 2 minutes. After that, move them to the wire rack. Let them cool.

Crispy Baked Chicken with Cheese

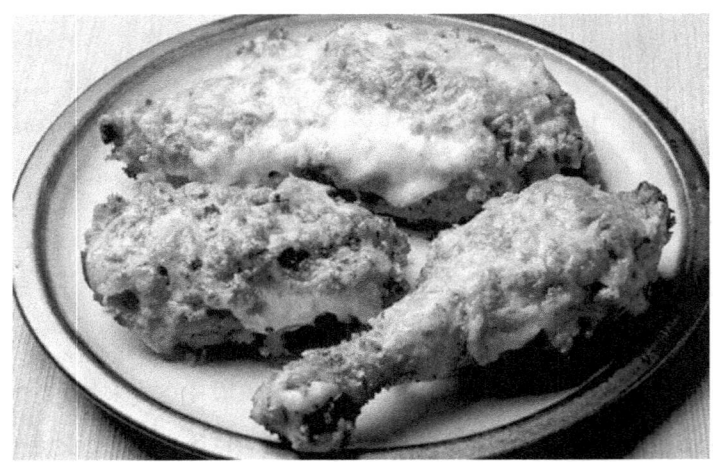

Ingredients

Whole chicken (in the form of cut parts): 1

Salt: According to taste

Lemon pepper: According to taste

Italian seasoning: According to taste

Bread crumbs (As required)

Eggs (beaten): 2

Coconut oil: 2 tablespoons

Butter: 2 tablespoons

Mozzarella cheese or shredded cheddar: 1 to 2 cups

Directions

1. Marinate chicken with lemon pepper, Italian seasoning, and salt. Toss the chicken pieces so that you can mix them evenly. Refrigerate this chicken for an hour or until needed.
2. Now, preheat your oven to a temperature of 375 degrees Fahrenheit.
3. Meanwhile, take a small bowl, and beat eggs in it. Also, take out the bread crumbs, and place them on a separate bowl. When the eggs have been beaten, dip each

piece of chicken individually in them. After that, roll it in to the bread crumbs for coating, and place it on a large-sized glass pan. Repeat the procedure for each piece of chicken.

4. Now, put a bit of butter and coconut oil on each of the chicken pieces. Make sure that you use 2 tablespoons of both coconut oil and butter when spreading them on all the chicken pieces.

5. Place all the chicken pieces in the preheated oven. Bake them for about 30 to 45 minutes, or till the chicken is completely cooked.

6. After this, take the chicken pieces out from the oven. Top them with the shredded cheese, and return them to oven.

7. Now, change the temperature to 450 degree Fahrenheit, and bake the chicken pieces for another 5 to ten minutes. Here, make sure that you do not need to wait for the oven to get preheated.

8. When the cheese appears brown, it means that the crispy chicken is ready to be served.

Coconut Pancakes

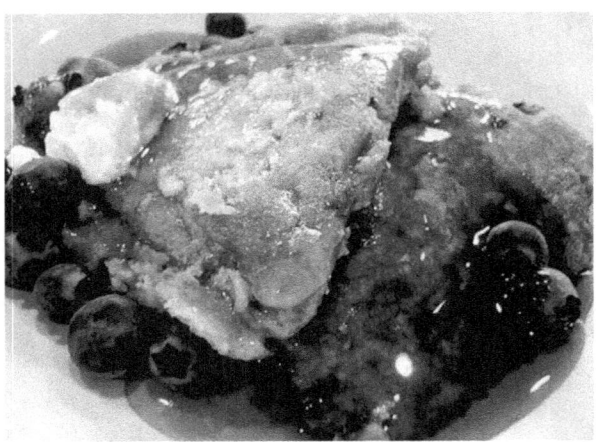

Ingredients

Banana: 1
Apple (small): 1
Flax seeds: 1 tablespoon
Nut milk or almond milk: ¼ cup
Coconut oil: 2 tablespoons
Coconut flour: 2 tablespoons
Rolled oats: 1/3 cup
Cinnamon: 1 pinch
Vanilla extract

Optional Ingredients as Add in's:

Baking soda: ¼ teaspoon
Baking powder: ¼ teaspoon
Nut milk/almond milk or water: ¼ cup (To be used only when the batter is too think or dry)

Directions

1. Take a blender, and blend banana, apple, flax seeds, and nut milk/almond milk in it. Once this is done, leave the mixture there for at least ten minutes. This way, flax seeds will be mixed well with the other ingredients. This will show the effect which is similar to beaten eggs.

2. To come up with creatively-prepared coconut pancakes, you can add the optional ingredients in the same mixture. Once this is done, mix them well till you see a smooth and even pancake mixture.

3. Now, take a pan, and pour two tablespoons of coconut oil in it. After heating it, pour the appropriate amount of pancake mixture on it, and fry each side for about four minutes while flipping the side accordingly.

4. Add two more tablespoons of coconut oil in the same pan. Fry the pancakes for about three minutes or till done. Garnish with your favorite fruit.

Appetizer Recipes

Apple Pie with Coconut Cream

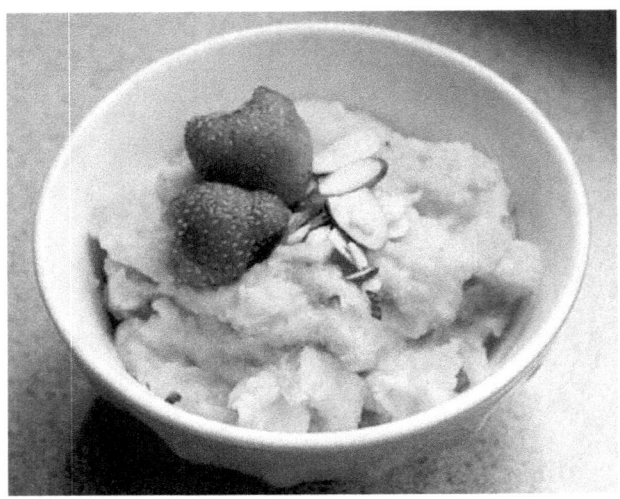

Ingredients

Apple juice: ½ cup
Apple (finely chopped): 1
Banana (large, roughly chunked)
Coconut cream concentrate: 2 heaped tablespoons
Shredded coconut: 2 tablespoons
Cinnamon
Nutmeg
Sea salt: 1 pinch

Directions

1. Take a small-sized saucepan, and pour apple juice in it. Start boiling it while adding all the remaining ingredients in it. Cover the pan, and cook it over medium heat till this mixture starts melting together. This will take about 1 to 2 minutes.

2. Remember that you are required to make the mixture thick, which is possible only if you make the right use of the coconut cream concentrate. So, continue cooking the mixture till you get the desired thickness.

3. When this is done, pour the apple pie mixture onto a bowl. Let it cool at room temperature, and then top it with fruits, nuts, or coconut.

Coconut Cheese Crackers

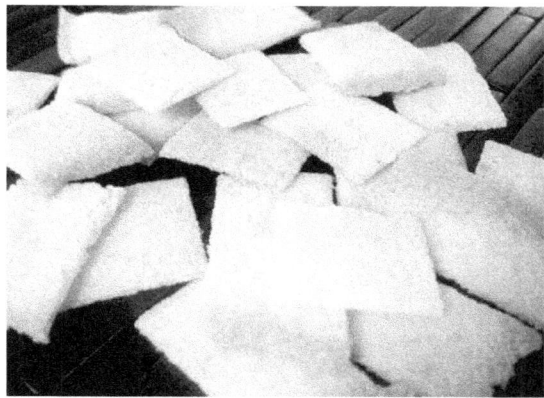

Ingredients

Coconut flour: ½ cup
Egg: 1
Butter: 2 tablespoons
Cheddar cheese (shredded): 1 ½ cups
Salt: 1 pinch

Directions

1. Preheat your oven at the temperature of 400 degree Fahrenheit.

2. Take a high-power food processor or blender, and blend all the ingredients in it together till they are combined well.

3. Now, spread the cracker batter on a cookie sheet lined with parchment paper. Place one more parchment paper over the mixture, and spread the batter by using the rolling pin. Pull off this parchment paper gently.

4. Bake the crackers for ten minutes. Once you have baked them, take them out, and give them the shape by cutting them with a pizza cutter, or a knife.

5. Now, put the crackers back in the oven, and bake them again till they are crisp and lightly brown. This will take about five to ten minutes.

Split Pea and Coconut Soup

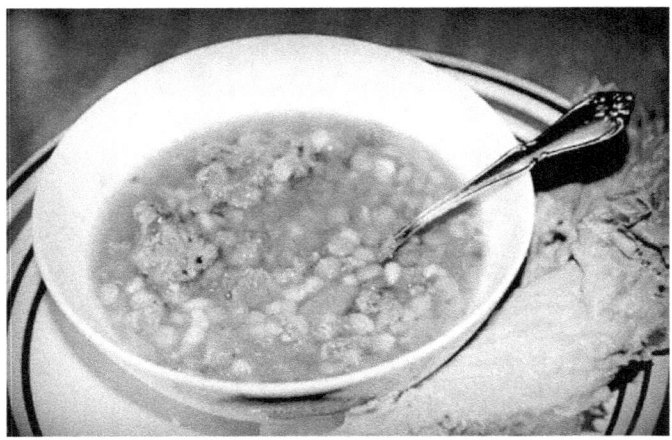

Ingredients

Coconut oil: 2 tablespoons
Celery (chopped): ½ cup
Carrots (chopped): 1 cup
Onions (chopped): 1 cup
Sea salt: 2 teaspoons
Split peas (green, rinsed well): 1 ½ cup
Vegetable broth: 4 cups
Ground turmeric: 1 teaspoon
Cumin seed: 1 teaspoon
Black pepper: 1 teaspoon
Ground beef (seasoned and cooked by using sausage seasoning): 1 pound

Directions

1. Take a large-sized pot, and add 2 tablespoons of coconut oil in it. Set this over medium heat.

2. When the coconut oil has been heated for cooking, add carrots, onions, celery, and salt in it. Cook these vegetables till the onions are semi-transparent. This will take about five to seven minutes.

3. Now, add broth, split peas, cumin, turmeric, and pepper into it. Combine all the seasonings by stirring them. Meanwhile, turn its heat from medium to high. Bring this dish to boil. When it starts boiling, reduce its heat, cover the pan, and simmer the dish for about an hour. Stir occasionally. Now, add the cooked and seasoned ground beef in the same pan. Simmer it for about ten minutes. Split pea and coconut soap is ready to serve.

Lunch Recipes

Coconut Rice

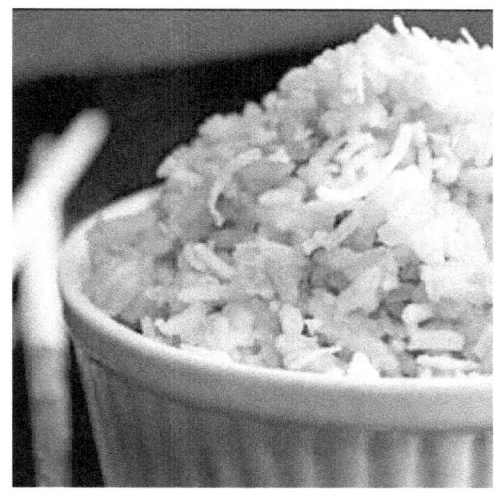

Ingredients

Coconut oil: 2 tablespoons
Brown rice: 3 cups
Water: 6 ½ cups
Fresh lime: 1
Toasted coconut (dried and unsweetened): ½ cup

Directions

1. Take a medium-sized pan, pour coconut oil in it, and heat it. Now, pour rice in it, and cook it till the color of rice darkens. Meanwhile, stir rice constantly.

2. Pour 2 cups of water at a time, and keep cooking the rice. Turn the heat from medium to high for boiling the rice. Leave the pan uncovered.

3. When the rice has been swelled, cover half of the pan and cook it for about ten to fifteen minutes. After that, cover the entire pan while turning the heat over low temperature. Let it simmer till the rice has become tender.

4. Fluff the rice with fork. Squeeze fresh lime on the top. You can also add a bit of butter on the top of rice. Garnish the delicious brown rice with dried and unsweetened toasted coconut. Coconut rice is ready to be served with fish or chicken.

Fried Coconut Zucchini

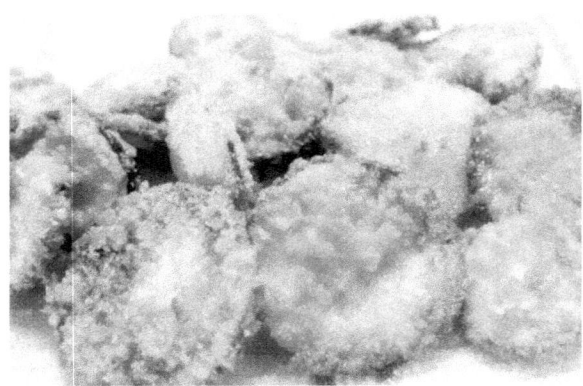

Ingredients

Coconut oil: 3 tablespoons (For frying)
Eggs (beaten): 2
Zucchini (thinly sliced): 2 cups
Coconut flour: ½ cup
Parmesan cheese (grated): ½ cup
Salt: 1 teaspoon

Directions

1. Take a frying pan, and pour coconut oil in it. Heat it over low to medium heat.

2. Meanwhile, take a medium-sized bowl, and add the eggs in it. Beat them lightly. You will need this egg mixture to dip with zucchini slices.

3. Now, take another bowl, and add Parmesan cheese, coconut flour, and salt in it. Mix these ingredients well. The flour mixture is ready.

4. Dip slices of zucchini into the egg mixture. After that, place the dipped slices in the flour mixture for coating. Make sure that you coat the zucchini slices well.

5. Fry these flour-coated zucchini slices till they turn golden brown. This will take about three to five minutes per side.

6. When you are done with frying them, place them on a plate covered with a paper towel. This will absorb the extra oil from the fried zucchini. Fried coconut zucchini is ready to serve.

Ginger and Plum Crisp With Flaked Coconut

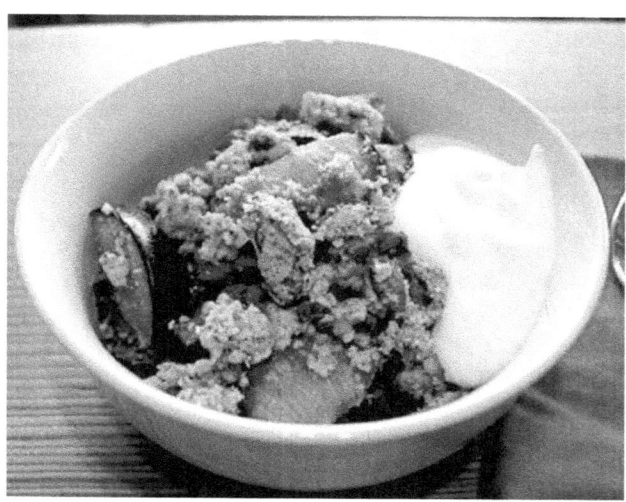

Ingredients

Almond flour: 1 cup
Flaked coconut (unsweetened): ½ cup
Cinnamon: 1 teaspoon
Salt: 1 pinch
Honey: 1 tablespoon
Coconut oil: 5 tablespoons
Pecans (chopped): ½ cup
Red plums (sliced and pitted): 2 ½ pounds, i.e. 8 medium-sized plums
Heavy cream: 2 tablespoons
Vanilla extract: 1 teaspoon
Crystallized ginger (chopped): 3 tablespoons

Directions

1. Preheat your oven to the temperature of 375 degrees Fahrenheit. Meanwhile, take a baking pan of 6X10 inches, and grease it. Now, take a small-sized mixing bowl, and add flaked coconut, almond flour, honey, cinnamon, and salt. Mix all these ingredients well. After this, stir in coconut oil (in its melted form), and then the pecans. Mix everything again till you get a smooth topping.

2. Take sliced plums, and spread them in the greased baking dish. Drizzle with vanilla and cream. Now, sprinkle the crystallized and chopped ginger evenly on the top of it. Once this is done, spoon the prepared topping over sliced plums.

3. Bake it for about 35 minutes, or till the topping becomes lightly brown. Serve the dish with whipped cream.

Dinner Recipes

Coconut Tuna Steaks with Lime

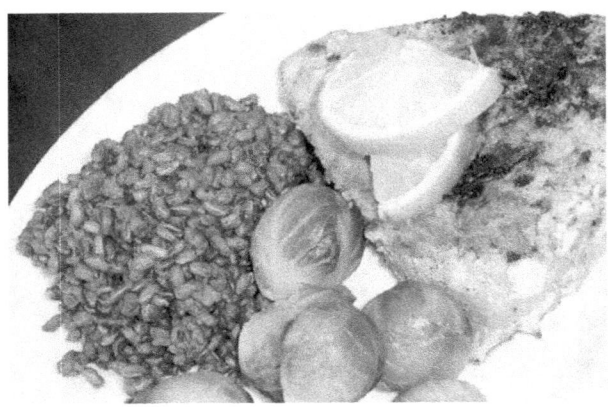

Ingredients

Olive oil: 2 ½ tablespoons
Seafood seasoning: 1 ½ tablespoons
Coconut cream concentrate: 1 ½ tablespoons
Organic limes: 2
Tuna steaks: 2
Coconut oil: 2 ½ tablespoons

Directions

1. First of all, wash the tuna steaks well. After that, rub both the sides of each steak with seafood seasoning and olive oil to coat.

2. Now, take a medium-sized bowl, and pour freshly squeezed juice of lime and coconut cream concentrate in it. Mix the two ingredients well till the mixture becomes creamy and smooth. The coconut-lime mixture is ready.

3. Apply this mixture as a coating for each side of the steaks. Its layer should be thick. As you coat one side of the steak with this coconut-lime mixture, wait for some time to make it hard. Once you see a hard layer on the first side of the steak, flip the side, and apply the mixture on the other side in the same manner.

4. When you are done with the coating, allow the steaks to be marinated for at least 10 minutes. This will help in terms of absorbing the flavors.

5. Now, take a skillet, and coat it with coconut oil. Preheat the skillet over medium temperature for five minutes. Cook the steaks well. The time required for its cooking may vary because it entirely depends on the steaks' thickness. However, in general, it will take about 2 to 3 minutes for each side of tuna steak to be cooked till desired doneness.

6. Flip the steaks carefully as it will retain the coconut coating. Once they are dome, garnish with lime and other vegetables. Coconut tuna steaks with lime are ready to be served.

Coconut and Curry Shrimp

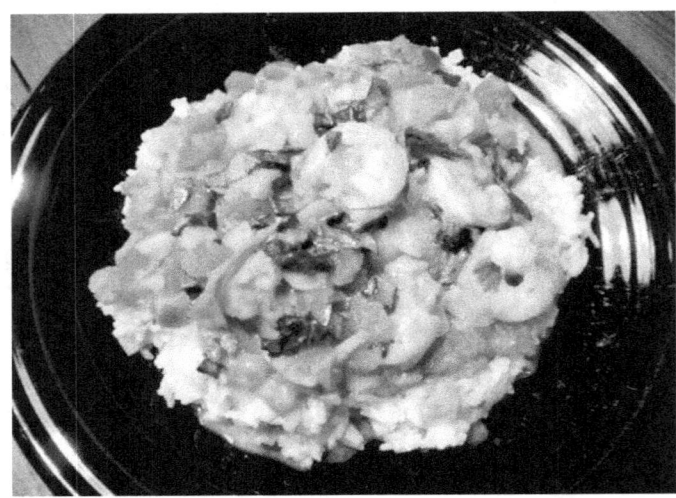

Ingredients for Shrimp

Shrimp (peeled and deveined): 1 pound
Red onion (sliced): 1
Coconut oil: 1 tablespoon
Thai curry paste (red or green): 1 to 2 teaspoons
Roasted tomatoes (diced and drained): 1 can, i.e. 14 oz.
Lime juice: 1 tablespoon
Fish sauce (optional): 1 teaspoon
Coconut milk: ½ cup
Basil (chopped): ¼ cup

Ingredients for Rice:

Basmati rice (uncooked): 1 cup
Coconut milk: 1 cup
Water: 1 cup
Coconut oil: 1 tablespoon
Salt: ½ teaspoon

Directions

1. Sauté onion and shrimp in one tablespoon of coconut oil till the shrimp become opaque. Stir in Thai curry paste. Cook it for a minute.

2. Now, stir in lime juice, fish sauce, and tomatoes. Heat this mixture to boiling. When this is done, simmer for a minute.

3. Now, stir in basil and ½ cup of coconut milk. Heat the dish in low temperature till it is hot. The shrimp mixture is ready. Keep it aside while keeping it warm.

4. Combine all ingredients of rice in a large-sized sauce pan. Heat them to boiling. When you see it boiling, reduce the temperature from high to low heat. Simmer it for about fifteen minutes or till the rice has become tender. Coconut rice is ready. You can serve the delicious shrimp as the topping over the coconut rice.

Green Fried Tomatoes

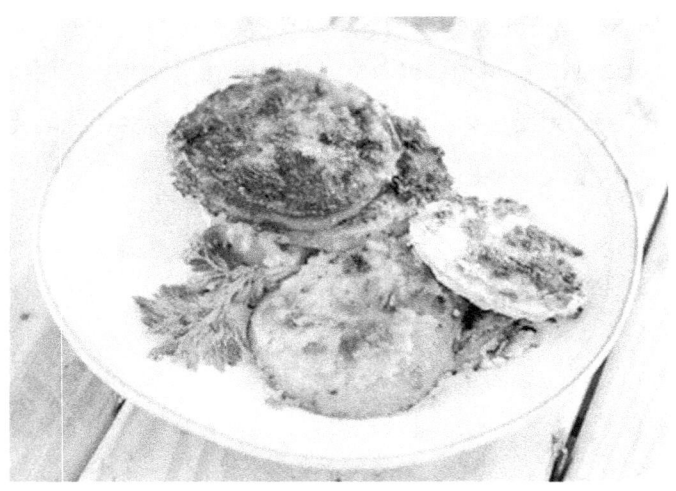

Ingredients

Coconut flour: ½ cup
Salt: ¼ teaspoon
Pepper: ¼ teaspoon
Paprika (optional): ¼ teaspoon
Egg (lightly beaten): 1
Green tomato (large-sized, in the form of slices of ¼ inch size)
Coconut oil: 2 to 4 tablespoons

Directions

1. Take a deep bowl, and combine coconut flour, pepper, salt, and paprika in it. The coconut-flour mixture is ready.

2. Now, take another bowl, add the egg in it, and beat it. Dip in tomato slices, and then dip them into this coconut-flour mixture.

3. Take a skillet, and heat it for about five minutes. Make sure that the temperature of the skillet is set over medium to high heat. Now, add coconut oil. Fry the tomato slices until they are light brown. This will take about two to three minutes for each side of the tomato slice. Fried green tomatoes are ready to be served.

Dessert Recipes

Coconut and Butter Truffles

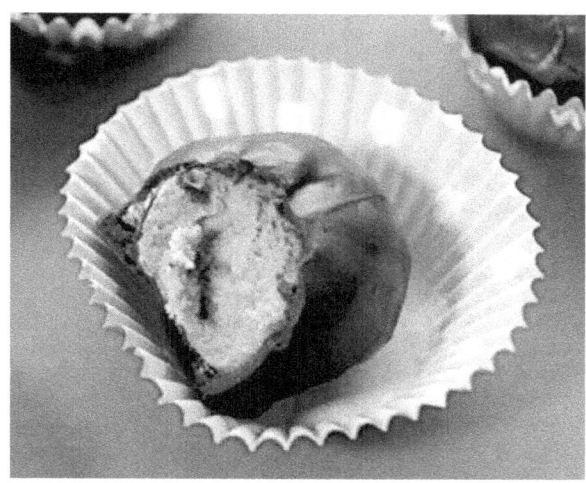

Ingredients

Coconut cream concentrate (softened/warmed): ½ cup
Coconut cream: 1/3 cup
Tea powder (matcha tea): 1 ½ tablespoons
Honey: 4 tablespoons
Dark chocolate or cocoa: For rolling and dipping

Directions

1. Take a medium-sized bowl, and pour the coconut cream concentrate and the coconut cream in it. Mix both the ingredients well. Now, add matcha tea along with honey. Mix it again. Truffle filling is ready.

2. Refrigerate this truffle filling for fifteen minutes, or till you think that it has become firm to be rolls into balls. Now, take out this filling, and roll it by using your hands. Come up with small rounds by using 1 tablespoon of the mixture to be filled in each truffle.

3. When you have rolled the truffles, sprinkle some cocoa, and then keep them in the refrigerator. You can also dip the truffles in dark chocolate. To do this, keep them in the refrigerator beforehand.

4. To dip truffles in dark chocolate, break up the chocolate, while heating it gently in low flame till it has been melted completely. Now, dip these truffles in the chocolate. After that, place the dipped truffles on the waxed paper and cool them. Coconut and butter truffles are ready to be served.

Coconut Lemon Meringues

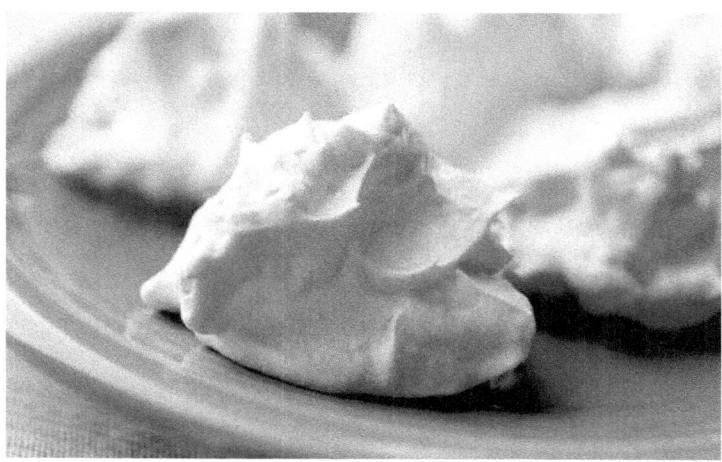

Ingredients

Egg whites: 4
Tartar cream: ¼ teaspoon
Powdered sugar: 1 cup
Vanilla extract: ½ teaspoon
Lemon zest: 1 to 2 teaspoons
Dried coconut (shredded)

Directions

1. Preheat your oven to the temperature of 250 degrees Fahrenheit. Also, line 2 cookie sheets along with the parchment paper.

2. Now, take a large-sized bowl, and beat the egg whites with tartar cream at high speed. Blend them well till you see a soft mixture.

3. Sprinkle sugar slowly (two tablespoons at one time) in the egg and tartar mixture while beating the whole mixture at a high speed. Keep adding the sugar gradually. After you have added and blended the mentioned quantity of sugar, it is time to beat in lemon zest and vanilla extract in the same mixture.

4. Beat it till you see the glossy and stiff peaks of meringue.

5. Drop the rounded spoonfuls of meringue onto the cookie sheets you had been prepared. Keep a distance of 1 inch between them. Now, sprinkle some shredded coconut.

6. Bake for fifty to sixty minutes, or till the dessert is dry when you touch it. Remove from oven, and cool it. Coconut lemon meringues are ready to be served.

CHAPTER 10

How to Make Fresh Coconut Oil At Home

What is better than to use coconut oil that has been made at your home? Preparing coconut oil at home does not only give you a clear idea that the oil is free from any harsh chemicals, it gives you the motivation to solve many of your problems. So, whether it is about using the same oil to get rid of skin infections, or beautifying your face, you can use coconut oil made by yourself.

It is quite easy to learn how to make it. Here are some of the basic instructions you need to follow:

1. Buy a coconut from the market, and split it by using a sharp ax. Make sure that you purchase a brown, mature coconut instead of a green one.

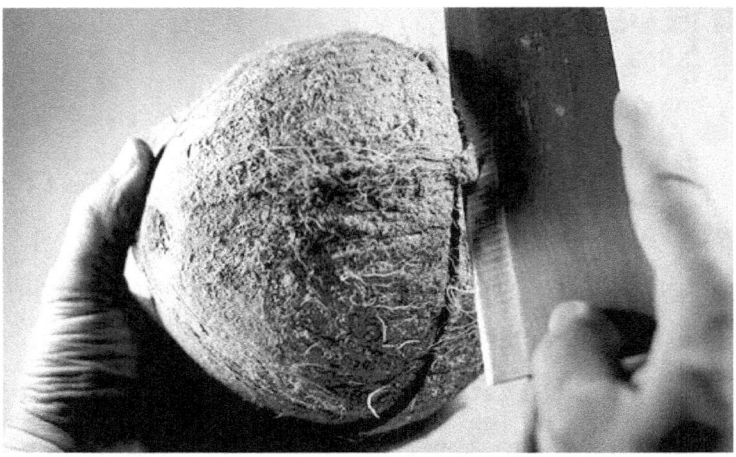

2. Once you have cut it into half, scrap all the coconut stuff from its shell. To do this, you will need a sharp knife or a metal spoon.

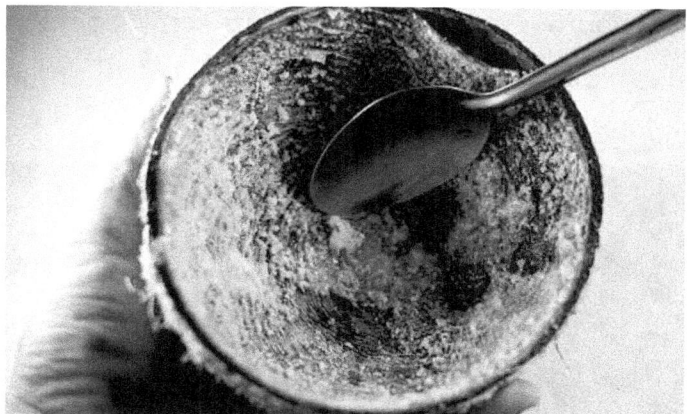

3. Cut this coconut stuff/meat in the form of chunks.

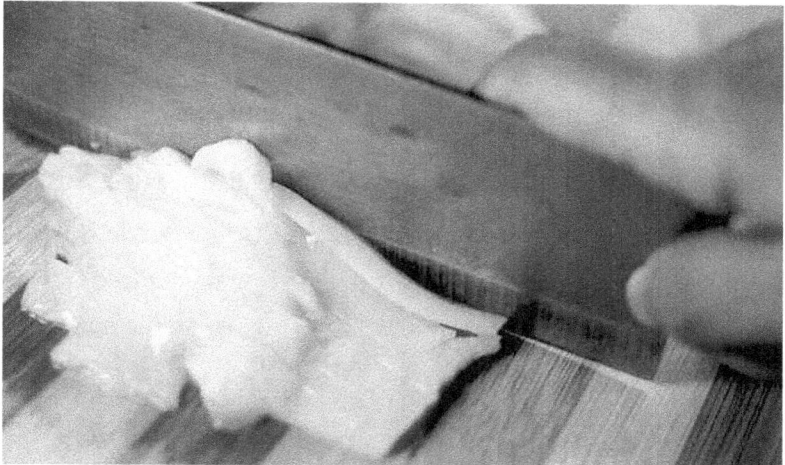

4. Place these chunks into a blender.

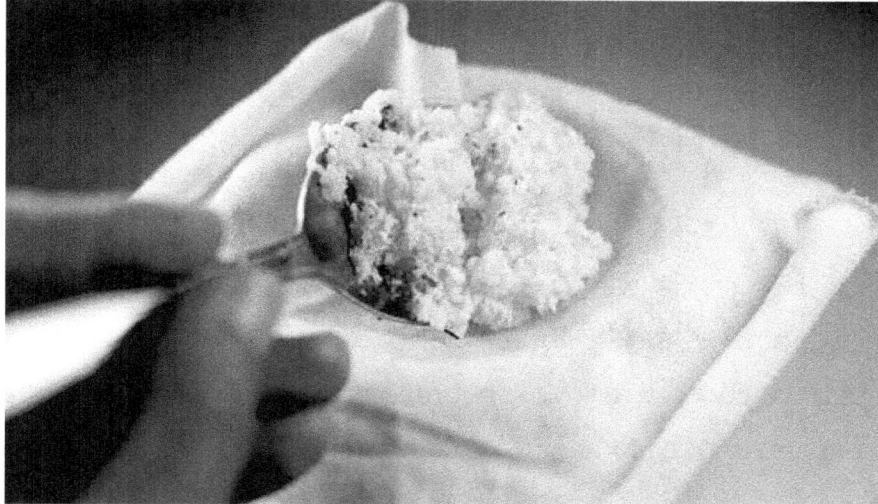

5. Process the coconut chunks over medium speed. Blend the pieces till they are well shredded. To make the blending easier, add a bit of water in the blender.

6. Now, take a jar, and put a cloth over it. Pour some portion of the grinded coconut mixture onto this cloth. After that, wrap the same cloth around this coconut mixture while squeezing the coconut milk into this jar.

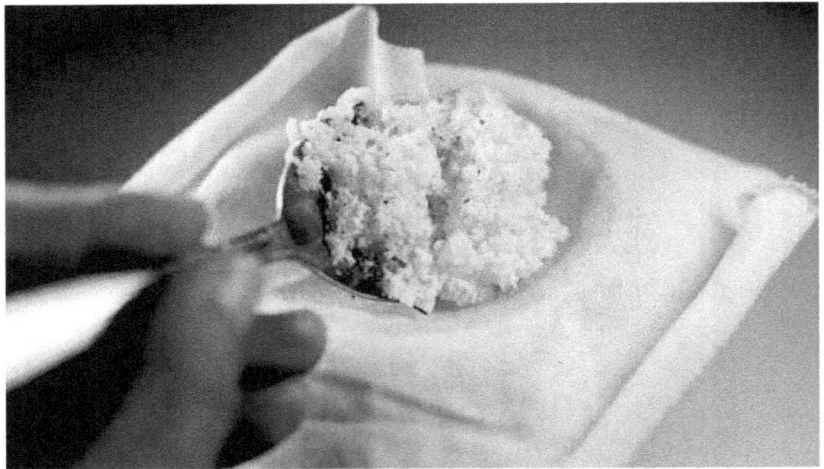

7. Remember to squeeze hard. This way, you will be sure that you are able to add each drop of coconut milk into the jar. Repeat the process till you have successfully transferred all the coconut mixture into the jar.

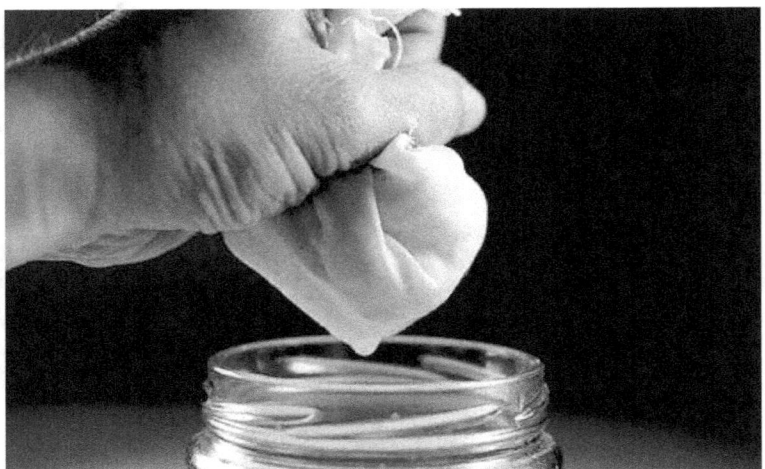

8. More than half of the work is done! All you need to do now is to leave this jar unattended, at least for 24 hours. The coconut mixture will take some time to set. As it is set, the coconut milk will separate from coconut oil. Additionally, you will see a prominent layer of coconut curd appearing on the top.

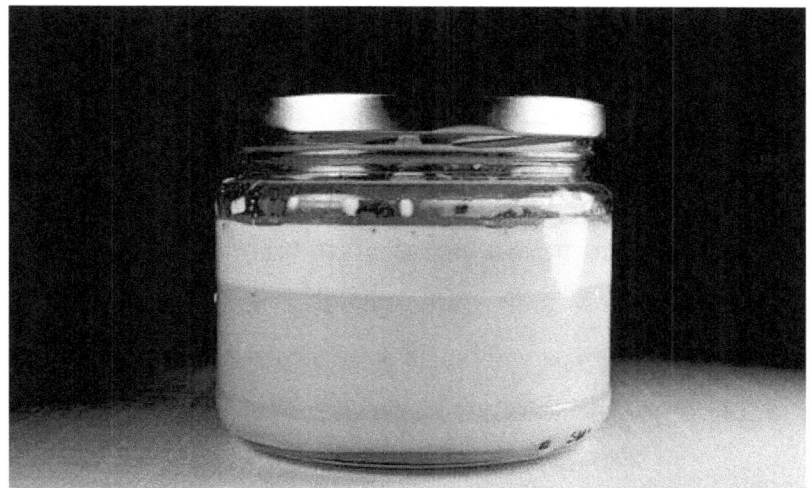

9. To make the curd more visible, put the jar in the refrigerator. After that, separate the curd with the help of a spoon. Now, the only thing left is pure coconut oil. You can use it and benefit from it.

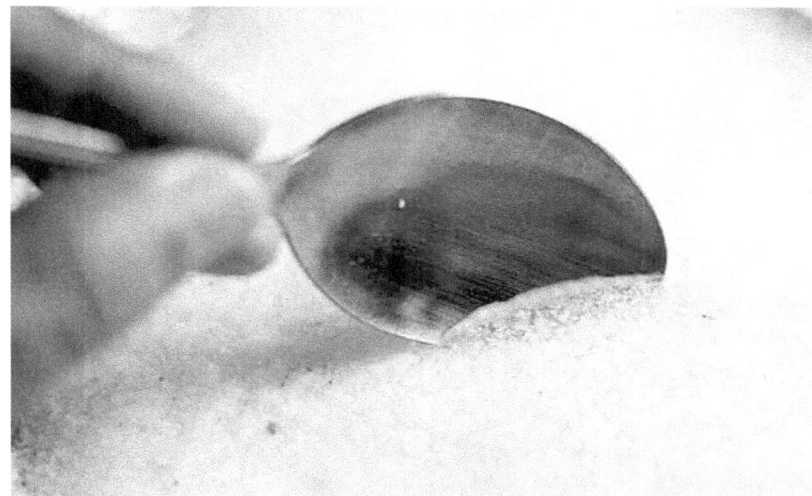

Final Word

Now that you have read all about coconut oil, its benefits, various uses, the different dishes to be prepared from coconut oil, and even the easiest way to prepare it at home, this special oil is definitely worth adding to your daily lifestyle. Once you start using coconut oil for your hair care, skin care, health, or simply in cooking, you will be exploring its benefits on your own. This is when you will analyze why coconut oil is considered unique as compared to other kinds of oil.

www.ingramcontent.com/pod-product-compliance
Lightning Source LLC
Chambersburg PA
CBHW081122280526
45787CB00007B/2939